Jing Jin Yoga

Stretches for the Fascia Combining the Asanas of Yoga with the Tendinomuscular Pathways of Chinese Medicine

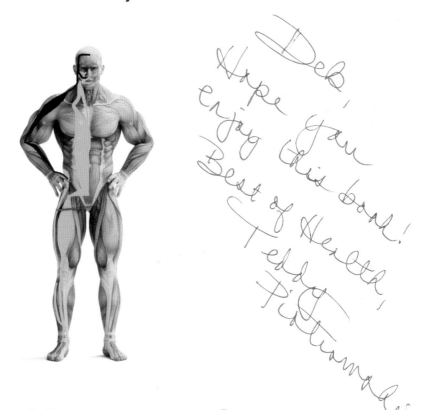

Deborah Valentine Smith

Barbara "Teddy" Piotrowski

Nourishing Practice for Self-Care

JINGJIN YOGA

Stretches for the Fascia Combining the Asanas of Yoga with the Tendinomuscular Pathways of Chinese Medicine

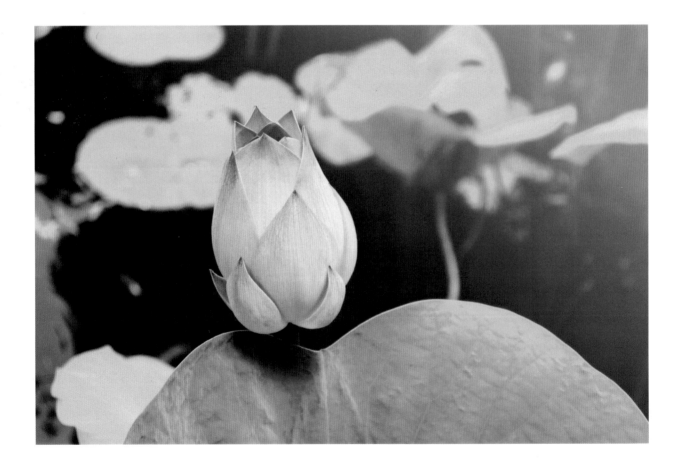

Contents

Preface to *JingJin* Yoga...1

Chapter One: *JingJin* and the Fascia....................................3

Chapter Two: The *JingJin* and the Immune System..........7

Chapter Three: The Mind/Body Connection......................11

Chapter Four: How to Use this Book 15

    JingJin Hand/Foot Pairs   16

    How to Use the Stretches   17

    The Approach: Take it Slow!   18

    The Contentment Formula   18

    Balance of Yin and Yang   18

    Before you Stretch, Focus the Mind   20

    Doing the Stretches   21

    Simple Diagrams of the Six *JingJin* Stretches   22

Chapter Five: Yang *JingJin* Stretches 25

    General Instructions   27

    Small Intestine/Bladder – *Tai Yang JingJin*   28

    Warrior I   29

    Triple Warmer/Gall Bladder – *Shao Yang JingJin* 32

    Warrior II/Side Angle   33

    Large Intestine/Stomach – *Yang Ming JingJin* 36

    Locust Pose   37

Chapter Six: Yin *JingJin* Stretches 41

    General Instructions   43

    Lung/Spleen – *Tai Yin JingJin*   44

    Reclining Bound Angle I   45

    Pericardium/Liver – *Jue Yin JingJin*   48

    Reclining Bound Angle II   49

    Heart/Kidney – *Shao Yin JingJin*   52

    Reclining Bound Angle III   53

Appendix I: Sequence Review 57

    JingJin Stretches - Version I   58

    JingJin Stretches - Version II   60

Appendix II: Traditional Chinese Medicine 62

Appendix III: Link to *JingJin Yoga* Videos 64

Bibliography 65

Related Internet Links 65

Acknowledgements...66

Graphics/Photo Credits 67

About the Authors 68

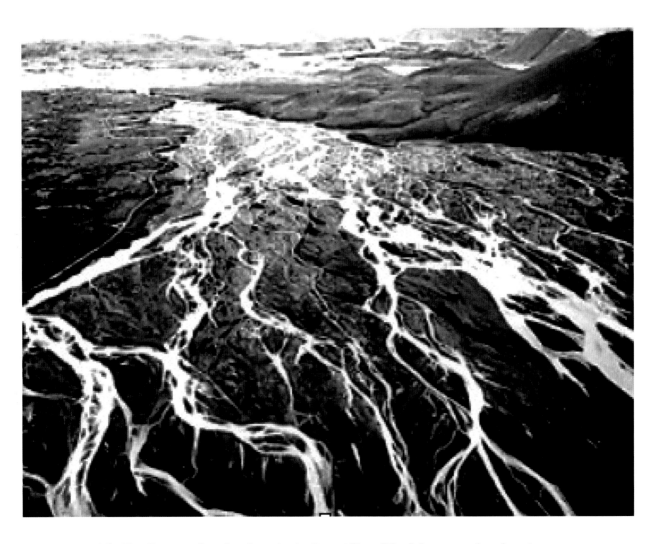

The JingJin are related to the principal meridians like deltas are related to rivers. They are branches that create broad zones in the superficial fascia to nourish muscles, tendons, and ligaments and form a protective layer of Wei Qi.

Preface to
JingJin Yoga

By Deborah Valentine Smith

THE JINGJIN ARE PART OF THE ENERGY TRANSPORTATION SYSTEM MADE UP of meridians and channels described by Chinese Medicine. The most familiar channels are the 12 "organ meridians," that flow through the entire body, including the interior organs. The JingJin are branches of these principal pathways that nourish the muscles and superficial fascia along their route.

The word "*jin*" is usually translated as "sinew" or "fascia" and includes both muscle and tendon. "*Jing*" refers to channels, thus the English translation of "*jingjin*" as "tendinomuscular meridians." The trajectory of these energy channels deviates from the regular meridians of Chinese Medicine, which follow a distinct path like a river. (See Appendix II: The Principal Meridians of Chinese Medicine) The *JingJin* are more like deltas spreading in a broad zone up through the fascia to nourish muscles, tendons, and ligaments. The method I developed for treating the *JingJin* uses techniques from many forms of bodywork for stretching and opening the fascia, including shiatsu stretches and yoga postures. I found that conscious intention, or mental focus, greatly reduced the physical effort involved in the acupressure point work and stretches. Indeed, many manual therapists who have taken my courses have told me that these techniques accomplish at least the same effects as deep tissue work with much less effort.

It seemed to me that the slow, conscious movement disciplines like *Tai Chi*, *Qi Gong* and Yoga were also focused on opening restrictions in the fascia. This is very different from the focus in Western exercise on building muscle tissue. Teddy had the same idea when she took a workshop I was teaching on treating the *JingJin*, and being a Shiatsu practitioner as well as a yoga therapist, she made the same connections I had made. We got excited about pairing the ancient poses of Yoga with the *JingJin*. It was really no surprise to discover how closely they are aligned. It's the same body, no matter what the culture or geography.

We were fascinated by the process of exploring the ways that traditional *asanas* might address specific *JingJin* channels (and vice versa!). We found that by putting the knowledge of the trajectory of the channels together with the poses, a *JingJin* "tweak" of a yoga posture in what seemed like miniscule ways produced an immediate improvement in results. The result of our combination of a *JingJin* map with a yoga pose is a "*JingJin* Stretch."

These deceptively simple stretches profoundly benefit the whole body in many surprising ways that, when done regularly, are cumulative and limitless. The "reset" and realignment of the fascia can include, among other effects, reduction of tension and discomfort, support of the function of the immune system and reduction of stress and depression (See Chapter 1: "*JingJin* and the Fascia" and Chapter 2: "*JingJin* and the Immune System"). Because they work with the energetic pathways, the effects of the *JingJin* Stretches are greatly enhanced when combined with mental focus on the desired effect (See Chapter 3: "The Mind/Body Connection). Therefore, the instructions for the stretches include the accompanying focus of the mind.

I'm sure that experienced yoga practitioners have discovered these adjustments in the same way that experienced and effective bodyworkers naturally work with the opening of the fascia by "feel." We hope this booklet will contribute to that knowledge and provide an additional practical theory to expand its application. It is the result of our explorations to date. We have tested the techniques with yoga instructors, bodyworkers, clients and family members, who agree with us about their effectiveness. We hope that this material brings ease and joy to you, whether you use it in your bodywork practice, yoga teaching, or for your self-care.

Chapter One:

JingJin and the Fascia

THE CONCEPT BEHIND THIS BOOK IS VERY SIMPLE. WE ARE LITERALLY HELD together by a ubiquitous network of connective tissue that wraps every part of the body and connects it to every other part. These layers of wrapping surround every type of tissue and structure in the body and connect them to everything else: bone to muscle, muscle to skin; organs to body walls and to each other. This wrapping keeps everything in place in relation to each other so that, for instance, the churning of the stomach doesn't cause it to migrate through the abdominal cavity. This wrapping tissue is collectively called *fascia*. It also carries the blood and lymph vessels and the nerves to all the tissues, so a restriction in the fascia has far-reaching effects.

Structure of Skeletal Muscle

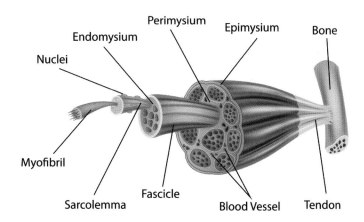

The Continuity of Fascia

The *endomysium* wraps each muscle fiber in a muscle cell.

The *perimysium* wraps muscle fiber bundles called "fascicles."

The *epimysium* wraps bundles of bundles to form the body of a muscle.

The *tendon* is formed by the meeting of all these fibers at the end, like the wrapping of a piece of hard candy. It connects to the *periosteum* that wraps the bone.

All these wrappings must be lubricated to allow for the movement that is crucial to the functioning of any tissue, yet they must be stable enough to provide support for the muscles, bones and organs and to hold them in the optimum position in relation to all the other structures. When fascia is not hydrated, structures that should be gliding over each other get stuck together. Imagine a sponge, supporting a heavy coffee mug. As it dries, the sponge takes on the contours of the mug. It resists efforts to bend and flex it to its original shape. Yet put the sponge in water, and as it absorbs the moisture, it returns to its original shape automatically, with no coaxing. You might say that it has "memory."

When fascia is not hydrated, the fibers get stuck together and distorted like a dry sponge. Yet like the sponge in water, as fascia absorbs the moisture, it returns to its original shape.

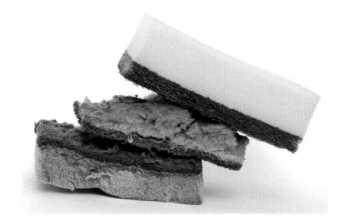

The same is true of fascia. It knows its shape in every nook and cranny of the body. Barring interference, it will return to that alignment of its fibers, and therefore to the best support for the optimum functioning of the tissues it wraps.

Clearly, if the fascia is stuck and distorted like the sponge, it will affect the functioning of whatever tissue it is wrapping. It can literally become twisted, and create pain and limited range of movement in our muscles and joints. This twisted wrapping also strangles crucial components like blood and lymph vessels, which usually keep a steady stream of fluid moving through the wrappings. Without that fluid, the fascia dries out even more and, in a vicious cycle, further impedes the delivery of the needed fluids.

How does the fascia get stuck? Obviously, trauma, especially if it results in scars, can distort the tissue. But by far the most common cause of "stuck fascia" is habitual muscle tension in reaction to stress. Some examples:

- You work long hours on a computer, holding your shoulders in place as you type. Over time, because of the lack of movement, which is needed to stimulate the flow of fluids, the fascia in your shoulders starts to stick to itself. To its credit, the mechanism is attempting to conserve energy by binding the position in place rather than using energy in continuous muscle contractions to hold the position. The lack of movement causes pain and the pain inhibits movement even more. Eventually you have what is called a "frozen shoulder", caused by dry, sticky fascia.

- You are injured in a car accident and have a large scar on your leg. As it is healing, that area is painful, and the scar tissue impinges on the blood and lymph vessels that facilitate healing. Because the stretching and limbering of the scar tissue that could return your leg to normal functioning is painful, you avoid movement, and the stickiness spreads.

- You have a good night's sleep. You are essentially immobile for 8 hours and when you awaken, since the normal movement that helps move fluid through the vessels and tissue has been minimal, you probably feel stiff and a little achy. If you don't get up and move and stretch, that discomfort will only continue, further impeding the needed circulation.

- You love your job, but you have a stressful relationship with your boss. You find yourself clenching your jaw in their presence in order not to blurt out how you really feel about their micro-managing. If the jaw muscles, like any muscles, are held in place long enough, the fascia will begin the process of sticking to itself, both from lack of lubrication, and from its effort to save your muscles the energy it takes to hold your jaw in place. Your jaw and then your neck and shoulders become progressively tighter, because muscles work in groups. When one is immobilized, it limits the movement of the other muscles connected to it.

So, what do you do about these problems? Turn back time to avoid the accident? Stop sleeping? Shout at your boss? These are not productive solutions. The good news is that, as we mentioned earlier, the fibers in the fascia remember the optimum position and alignment. They will respond eagerly to any assistance that can unstick them and return flexibility and flow. Stretching the muscles of the body in proper alignment with the direction of the fibers of the fascia is one way to accomplish that. But how do we know the proper alignment when we are stuck in distortions of it? The postures of yoga mimic that alignment. Using them to stretch the tissue not only loosens it but repositions it and reestablishes the flow of fluids. This supports the natural flexibility and strength that is characteristic of hydrated tissue, and by re-establishing the flow of blood, lymph, and Qi, it assists the nourishment and optimal functionality of the tissue.

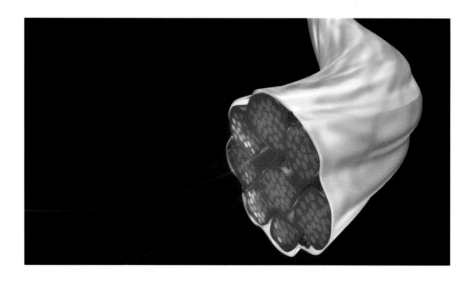

The principal energy channels of Chinese Medicine (see Appendix II) flow through the fascia along with the blood and lymph vessels and nerves. Current theory postulates that the "grain" of the fascia creates the network of the energy channels and subsidiaries that deliver the Qi to every cell in the body. So, when the meridians of acupuncture are distorted by blockages in the fascia, the adjacent tissue doesn't get the energy it needs to carry out its functions.

Yoga postures reestablish the natural alignment of the fascia that frees the channels of Qi and Blood that are described in the maps of Chinese Medicine. The maps, in turn, provide information about the direction of flow and the points along the trajectories that encourage the opening of the channels as the flows improve. The delivery of the Qi through the channels also provides the energy to move what is stuck. The stretches help to align the channels and re-establish the optimum delivery of the Qi and Blood where it is needed.

Chapter Two:

The *JingJin* and the Immune System

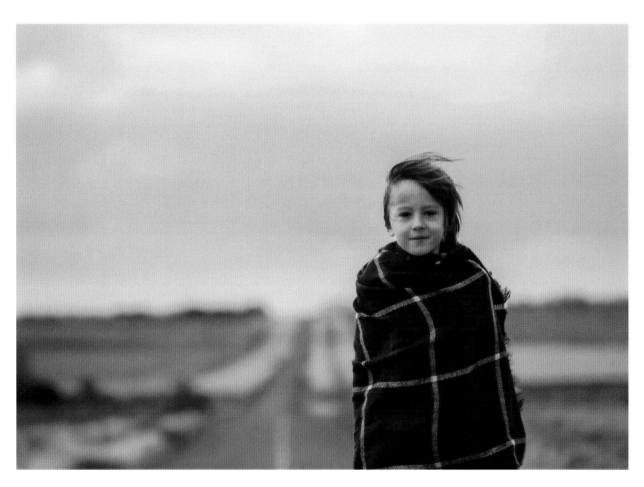

The Wei Qi flows through the JingJin, forming a protective wrapping of energy.

I T IS WELL-KNOWN IN WESTERN MEDICINE THAT OPTIMAL IMMUNITY CAN BEST be achieved through regular exercise, healthy sleep and a balanced diet. Relevant research shows that a regular yoga practice can (see link below):

- **lessen inflammation by downregulating the stress response**, which may reduce risk of infections;

- **improve sleep quality,** helping you feel rested and rejuvenated;

- **calm the nervous system** by going into the relaxation response more often, which in turn helps your organs to function optimally, giving your body greater capacity to fight invaders and heal;

- **improve immune function** (including mucosal and cell-mediated immunity, *key aspects of your body's first-line and sustained defenses,* particularly IL-1beta, IL-6, and TNF-alpha).

https://link.springer.com/article/10.1007/s10865-018-9914-y

How Can Yoga, Specifically *JingJin Yoga,* Improve Immune Function?

The skin plays an essential role in preventing excess "external influences" (wind, cold, damp, heat, micro-organisms, etc.) from overwhelming the body. It is the largest organ in the body and serves the immune system in crucial ways.

- It forms a physical barrier that maintains the integrity of the body.

- The deepest layer of the skin is composed of fascia that connects it to the underlying muscle. This basal layer also encloses blood vessels carrying white blood cells that protect against microscopic invasion from the surface.

- The basal layer also carries a protective wrapping of energy called *Wei Qi* (pronounced *Way Chee*). In acupressure theory, the *Wei Qi* flows in the "space between the skin and the muscles" (the basal layer of fascia) in designated pathways called the *JingJin.* These superficial channels come to the surface from the 12 principal meridians at the *Jing-Well* points on the fingers and toes (See Appendix II) and flow toward the torso, forming energetic "gloves," "galoshes," and "scarves" that allow us to interact harmoniously with nature.

- If there are restrictions in the fascia, the flow of the *Wei Qi* in the *JingJin* channels and of the blood in blood vessels is impeded.

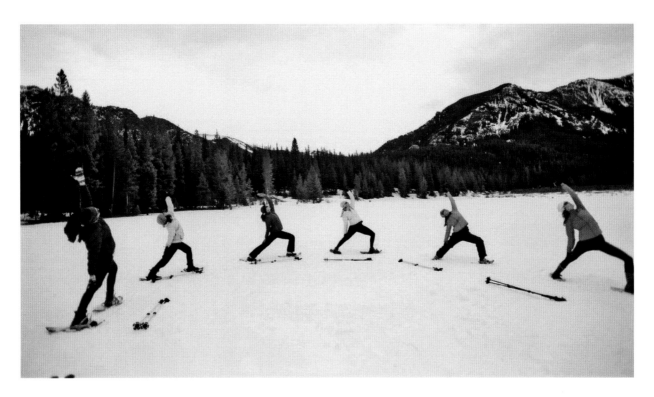

Flowing from the fingertips and toes toward the torso,
the Wei Qi *forms energetic "gloves," "galoshes" and "scarves."*

JingJin Yoga fine-tunes traditional yoga postures to match the trajectories of the *JingJin*, emphasizing the opening of the channels at the fingers and toes. As the postures align the fascial tracks with these crucial entry points, the inflowing *Wei Qi* opens the restrictions further. This combination makes the process almost effortless.

Exercise like Yoga keeps the fascial layer supple, thereby increasing the flow of the energetic *Wei Qi* and the flow of blood.

Follow your natural rhythms and begin a restorative practice like *JingJin Yoga*.

Chapter Three:
The Mind/Body Connection

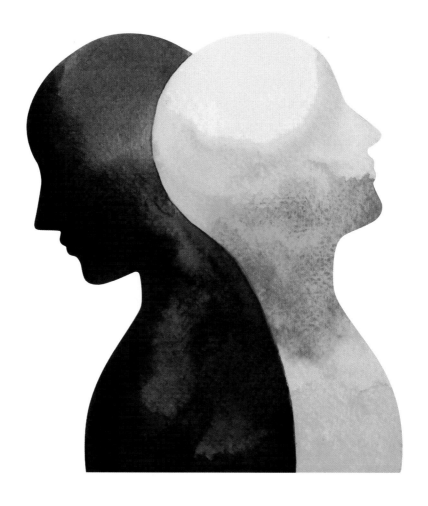

Blood follows Energy
Energy follows Mind
Mind follows Spirit
Spirit follows the Tao

The Taoist classics say:

Blood follows Energy
Energy follows Mind
Mind follows Spirit
Spirit follows the Tao

THE PRACTICES IN THIS BOOK WORK PARTICULARLY WITH THE FIRST TWO STATE-ments: "Blood follows Energy" and "Energy follows Mind." "Energy follows Mind" is a practical statement that checks out in Western science. When I decide to pick up the papers on my desk, it starts as an idea, in the mind, which translates into information sent from the brain through the spinal cord to the nerves that stimulate the muscles I need to do the action. At the same time, the capillary beds that feed those same muscles open to provide more raw materials that the cells need to produce the *energy* needed for the action. Therefore, the mind leads, and the energy follows.

This is easily demonstrated in voluntary movement of skeletal muscle, but we are now understanding more about how our thoughts also influence the so-called *involuntary* processes, like heartbeat, digestion, and emergency responses. Knowing this, it is possible that we can also *consciously* monitor our thought processes to ameliorate stress.

Working with energy flows, Yogis, Meditators and Asian Bodywork Therapists have noticed that intention has a profound effect on the movement of energy in the pathways, which in turn has a profound effect on the condition of the tissues. This is useful to remember. To improve the flow of *Qi* and blood and to enhance the flexibility of the tissue, we don't necessarily have to literally pull on the fascia. If we combine the influence of imagination, *especially including the feeling component,* on the energy at the subtle level, enhanced by the gentle positions of the stretches that align the fibers, the process is well on its way and it saves a lot of work.

This coupling of imagination and physical activity received a lot of interest several years ago during the Olympic high diving competition. Commentators noticed that members of the Chinese team, who were pull-ing down incredible scores, spent an unusually long time at the end of the diving board before they actually began the dive. It turned out that they were thoroughly imagining the feeling of the entire dive before beginning the physical move-ment. Given the extra preparation, their physio-logical responses were even more efficient.

So, you could translate this into how you do your stretches. You can do yoga or acupressure with a lot of effort and hard work because that's how we've been taught that things get accom-plished. The idea is that if you're not working hard

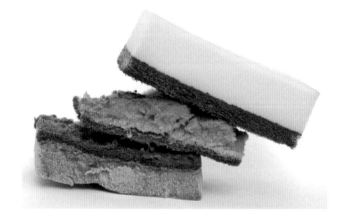

Fascia has memory, like the fibers in a sponge.

and challenging the limits of your body, you are not serious. With this work, however, we are asking you to try a new approach. Try working *with* the natural flow or position rather than trying to make it do something unusual.

Fascia has memory, like the fibers in a sponge. You can twist it, overstretch it or compress it, but as soon as you let go, if it is not actually torn or dried out, it will return to its original alignment. That pattern of fibers with their attachments is the optimum scaffolding for blood vessels and nerves and for holding organs in their most efficient position within the body. There is an ease of movement and grace that reflects the natural alignment and adaptability of the living, hydrated tissue. *Find that ease.* Try this method that starts with ease.

Here's an experiment you can try to demonstrate this principle of ease and efficiency to yourself. Start by paying attention to how your arm feels in the present moment, then grasp it at the wrist with the other hand. Pulling strongly down from the shoulder, create a substantial stretch in the upper arm and shoulder. Let go and take a moment to notice the effects of the stretch you've just done. Now move to the opposite arm and rather than *pulling* on it, just hold the wrist gently and *imagine the feeling* of pulling and stretching the arm without actual physical effort. Let go and take a moment to notice the effects of this imaginary stretch. How do they compare with the effects of the actual stretch?

You may find that the arm that you virtually stretched released at least as much or more than the other. This has to do partially with the body's response to a suggestion, rather than a physical challenge. With suggestion, it can respond in its own way, rather than succumb to a movement that is imposed on it that could possibly go too far. When pulled, the fascia goes only so far, but then does its job of holding things in place and preventing excessive movement that could create injury. Pulling on the body usually triggers protective resistance in the fascia, no matter how slight. We usually respond to that resistance by pulling on it more, thus creating more resistance and so on. When we offer an alignment *suggestion* instead, the tissue can try it out safely and find its own opening without needing the resistance. Applying this principal of "less is more" to yoga, we can move toward the stretch and imagine the feeling of it without forcing it and then follow the natural opening of the body as it tests the limits and then lets go.

This comes down to the balance between *doing* and *being.* There is a natural way that already exists. We don't need to create something new if we work with the potential that is inherent in our physical makeup. Sometimes outside assistance may be necessary to liberate adhesions caused by long time immobility and dehydration, but for the most part, the best effects come from gentleness and suggestion.

People with chronic fibromyalgia often request deep bodywork, because they subscribe to the "no pain, no gain" ethic. Unfortunately, fibromyalgia is often the result of just that same kind of unrelenting, demanding attitude. It may take a while for them to feel the subtle difference that results from work that doesn't trigger the body's protective response. Yoga *asanas*, when approached with gentleness and a sense of process, offer a way to return the fascia to its original alignment organically. The stretch is not a goal to be reached by any means necessary. Just because you *can* do something, it doesn't mean you have to. *The stretch is a guideline, a pathway toward alignment in the same way the meridian is the optimum pathway for the movement of* Qi. It shows us how to imagine a course from where the body is now back to its natural suppleness. *Any* movement along that trajectory is success. The posture helps the body remember the natural, original alignment in which the blood and energy flow smoothly through the tissue. When we pair the *JingJin* with the *asanas* and add conscious intention, there is minimal effort needed."

Chapter Four:

How to Use this Book

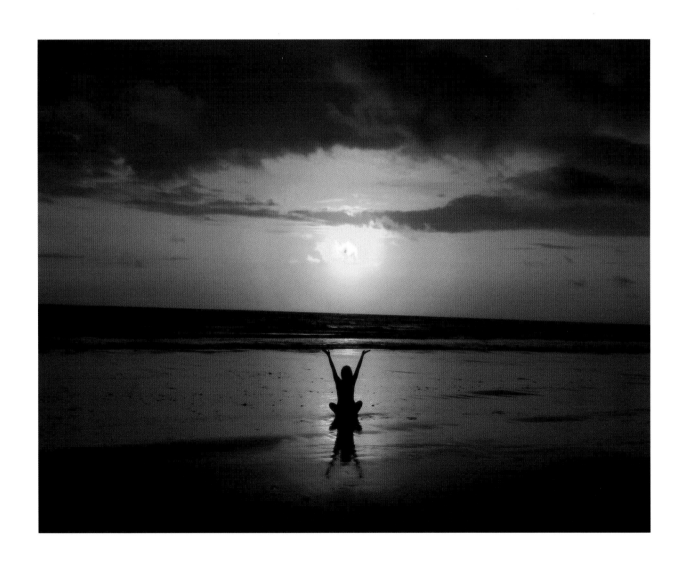

JingJin Hand/Foot Pairs

There are 12 *JingJin*, one branching from each of the 12 principal meridians of Chinese Medicine. (See Appendix II) When the six "hand" *JingJin*, which run from fingertips to torso or head, are combined with the six "foot" *JingJin*, which run from toes to torso or head, they follow a fascial track from head to toe. ***We've combined the six hand/foot pairs with the yoga postures that open the same fascial track to create the* JingJin *Stretch*.**

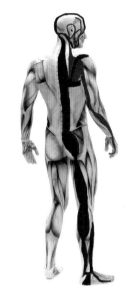

Tai Yang
Small Intestine/Bladder

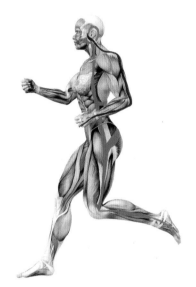

Shao Yang
Triple Warmer/Gallbladder

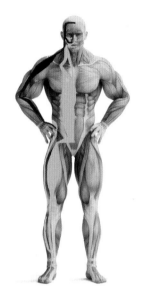

Yang Ming
Large Intestine/Stomach

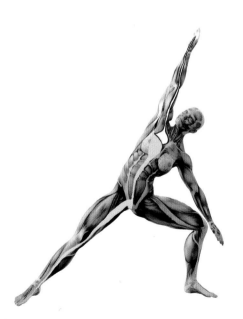

Tai Yin
Lung/Spleen

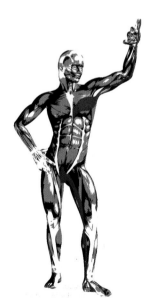

Shao Yin
Heart/Kidney

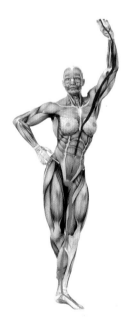

Jue Yin
Pericardium/Liver

How to Use the Stretches

Here are some simple ways to use these stretches. (If you want to delve further into the theories of Yin/Yang and the principal meridians, see Appendix II).

- **Start with self-assessment.** Look at the diagrams of the six *JingJin* to identify tracks that match what you are feeling in your body or what is calling for your attention.

- **Choose your approach:**

  - For a short session, choose one or two individual stretches that address a specific problem from Chapters 5 and 6.

  - Or, choose a general area: (Shown on the first page of Chapters 5 and 6)

    - Yang areas of the body, which are along the back and outside of the limbs

    - Yin areas, which are along the front and insides of the limbs

  - Or, do the whole sequence of six stretches outlined in Appendix I.

  - However you proceed, start with Version I of each stretch and move to Version II or III when they are accessible to you. Even if you need to begin with the modified position, the *JingJin* Stretch is very easy to duplicate, and you will find yourself progressing in a matter of days.

  - If you have specific areas of stiffness or pain, the *JingJin* maps can show what stretch will address it.

There is a section for each of the six *JingJin* Stretches that provides:

- A diagram of the trajectory of the *JingJin* pair

- A list of related muscles and tissues affected by the *JingJin* Stretch

- Simplified stick figures of the stretch

- A description of the related *JingJin* Stretch and the accompanying bodymind focus

- Photographs of a person doing the stretch

- Two or three versions of the stretch modified for different levels of flexibility

The Approach: Take it Slow!

Your physical condition is constantly in flux and adjusting to changes in your environment and activity, to physiological changes like injury, illness and aging, and to the responses of your emotional being to all of those influences. Your motivation for trying *JingJin Yoga* will affect how you approach it. You will gain the most benefit from this type of work if you take the time to check in with where you are in the present moment rather than where you used to be, want to be, or think you should be. Do this with conscious awareness. Let your body tell you what it is capable of *right now* and where it can go from here. Be kind. It will change from day to day.

The Contentment Formula

C = A/E

C = *Contentment*

A = What you can *achieve*

E = Your *expectations*

If you keep your expectations realistic without forcing your limits, you will be able to achieve them, which in turn will lead to contentment and the encouragement to continue and improve. For example, on a scale of 1-10, with 1 being the lowest & 10 being the highest, if what you can achieve ("A") is a 5, but your expectations ("E") are at 10, then your contentment is 5/10 or 50%. But, if what you can achieve is still a 5, but you now lower your expectations to a 5, then your contentment is now 5/5, which equals 100%. By lowering your expectations from 10 to a 5, you have guaranteed a positive outcome.

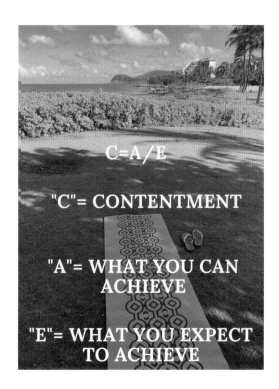

C=A/E

"C" = CONTENTMENT

"A" = WHAT YOU CAN ACHIEVE

"E" = WHAT YOU EXPECT TO ACHIEVE

Balance of Yin and Yang

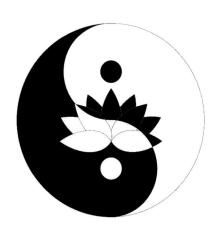

Yang. Some people, especially those in physically demanding environments like athletes, dancers and people who do manual work, expect to push through physical limitations. This meets the immediate physical demands of an activity, but can lead to injuries and further restrictions as the fascia protects the tissues by resisting the challenges. If you are this type of person, it will benefit you to pay more attention to the natural limits of your body and respect what it is telling you. You can give yourself the suggestion that you will get more results from these exercises if your goal is to *explore* the edge of your comfort zone, rather than to *break through* it.

Yin: People who are less physically active or more cautious, sometimes because of injury or pain, tend to settle for what is most comfortable without stretching their limits. If you are this type of person, it will benefit you to find the *edge* of that comfort zone and gently *extend* it. If you stay mindful, your body will let you know how far you can go, which will enhance your strength and, by releasing the restrictions in the fascia, increase your flexibility.

Remember, the goal is awareness.

- Be patient with yourself and stay in the present moment.

- Begin with Version I of the stretch and move on from there.

- Go slow, breathe, take it easy.

- Start at 75% of what you think you can do, then increase slowly, without forcing.

- Remember the balance of Yin and Yang: Look for your edge and stay just on the comfortable side of it. That is where you feel a pleasant stretch without excessive discomfort or pain. Let your body tell you when it's ready to extend the stretch.

- Start by centering and using abdominal breathing (see instructions below).

- When you are stretching, *inhale* as you lengthen, *exhale* as you release and open the fascia. The *release* is the important part.

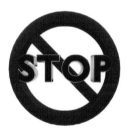

DON'T stop here.
You can use these techniques to fine tune any yoga *asana*.

Every movement of the body involves these fascial lines. Once you become familiar with the six ***JingJin* Stretches**, you can use the diagrams of the fascial lines served by the tendinomuscular meridians in this book to fine tune other poses. Identify the muscles involved in the pose and use the awareness of the *JingJin* as you practice it to open restrictions in the fascia. For instance, Downward Facing Dog stretches primarily the triceps, hamstrings and erector spinae. Looking at the list of muscles for each *JingJin, Tai Yang* is the closest match for this pose, so you would focus on the connection between the 5th finger and the 5th toe when doing the pose.

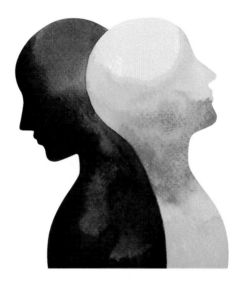

Before you Stretch, Focus the Mind

Energy follows Mind (See Chapter 3)

- **Engage the mind** and the visual and kinesthetic parts of the brain.

  ◦ **Look** at the maps of the *JingJin* and the pictures of the *JingJin* Stretches and notice how the stretch affects the *JingJin*.

  ◦ **Imagine the feeling of** doing each stretch before you start moving. Tune into the possibility of natural movement without strain. *Feel the connection between the specific finger and toe for the stretch. Imagine* the feeling of a string running through your body whose ends are your finger and toe. *Imagine* the feeling of reaching into the finger and toe and stretching them away from each other.

- **Direct the Breath and *Qi* with the Mind: *Hara* Breathing**. *Where the mind goes, the energy flows.*

  ◦ Imagine the feeling of your spine suspended from a bar above your head. Everything is hanging from that central pole. Imagine the feeling of the fascia releasing and opening.

  ◦ Watch your breath move in and out.

  ◦ Exhale to empty. As you breathe in, imagine the feeling of letting your belly open so the breath goes all the way down to the *hara* (the area just below the navel).

  ◦ As you breathe out, imagine the feeling of letting your belly deflate like a balloon letting out air.

  ◦ Breathe all the way down to the bottom of your *hara* and fill to the top of your chest, like filling a pitcher. When you exhale, deflate your chest first, keeping the *hara* expanded, and then empty the *hara*, like emptying a pitcher from the top down. This may take a little practice at first.

- As you continue breathing, imagine that with each inhale, you are taking in *prana* or *Qi*, which is energy. You can imagine it as light, sparkles, warmth, a vibration or even a tone that spreads all the way down inside to your *hara*. With the outbreath, imagine that the energy in your *hara* concentrates in the area below the navel. You are feeding the "golden stove" with the inhale and concentrating the energy inside it with the exhale.

- As the light gets brighter, the warmth spreads or the tone deepens, be aware that the universe is made entirely of *Qi*, which we can breathe in whenever we need it. We only need to let it in.

- Now find a place in your body that seems to be asking for attention. In your next exhale, imagine sending the concentrated energy from your *hara* to that place. Continue as long as you like. To finish, rub your hands together and place them over your eyes. Take a breath and open your eyes, letting them take in the warmth coming from your hands.

Doing the Stretches

Blood Follows Energy

Now the body is ready for you to **move into the *JingJin* Stretch.** You don't need to strain or work hard. *A gentle nudge toward the natural alignment is more effective than forcing it, so ease into it.*

- Center yourself. Ground yourself by feeling your connection to the earth. If you feel resistance, just stay centered and breathe.

- Start by doing a simple stretch between the finger and toe associated with the *JingJin* Stretch on one side. Play with the connection, experimenting with turning the hand and/or foot slightly to find the alignment that enhances the stretch.

- Repeat on the opposite side. Notice any difference between the two sides.

- As you assume the stretch, keep the relationship between the finger and toe. Find the stretch that feels like a natural connection. This is very important to prevent strain. If you feel resistance, lighten up, keep breathing!

- If you want to work on a particular problem area, look at the *JingJin* Stretch charts and pick the stretch that addresses that area.

- Start with the modified stretches with anchored support, which reduces tension.

- You can experiment with the order of the stretches. Some possibilities are:

  - Start with the Yang standing stretches, then the Yang stretch on the floor, and then the Yin stretches.

  - Reverse the order; start with the Yin/floor stretches and finish with the Yang.

  - Alternate Yin and Yang. (This means a lot of getting up and down from the floor.)

Simple Diagrams of the Six *JingJin* Stretches

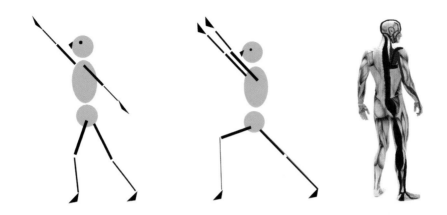

Tai Yang
Small Intestine/Bladder

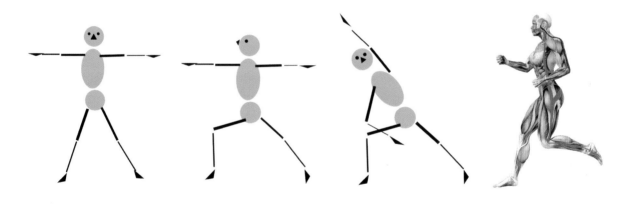

Shao Yang
Triple Warmer/Gall Bladder

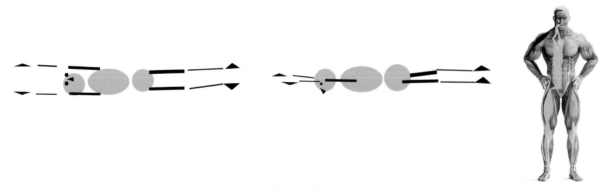

Yang Ming
Large Intestine/Stomach

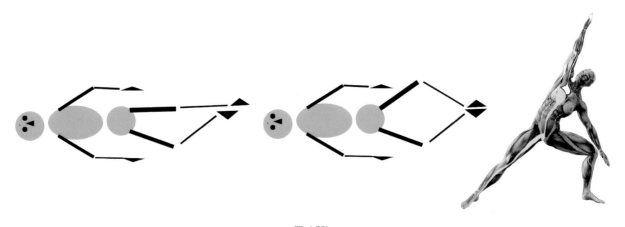

Tai Yin
Lung/Spleen

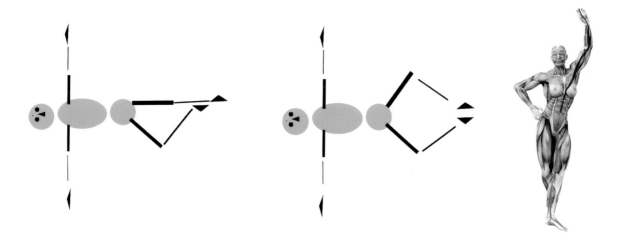

Jue Yin
Pericardium/Liver

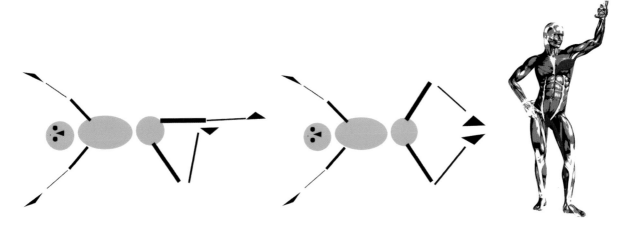

Shao Yin
Heart/Kidney

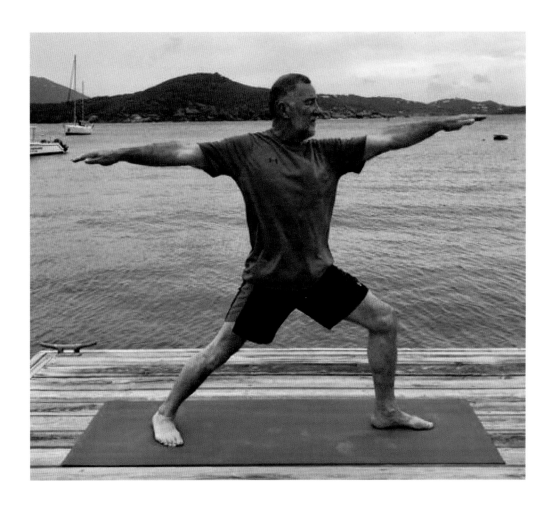

Chapter Five:

Yang *JingJin* Stretches

As You Begin:

Remember, the goal is awareness of your body.

Be patient with yourself and stay in the present moment.

Begin with **Version I** of the stretch.

Go slow, breathe, take it easy.

Remember the balance of Yin and Yang: Start at 75% of what you think you can do. Look for your edge and stay just on the comfortable side of it, where you feel that satisfying stretch without excessive discomfort or pain. Let your body tell you when it's ready to extend the stretch.

Breathing: Before starting the stretch, exhale to empty. During the stretch, *inhale* **as you lengthen,** *exhale* **as you release** and open the fascia.

The *release* **is the important part.**

Golden Rule
Less Is More!

THE YANG *JINGJIN* RUN ALONG THE BACK OF THE BODY AND THE OUTSIDE OF THE LIMBS.

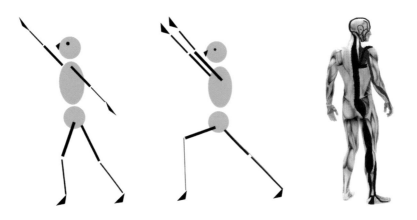

Tai Yang
Small Intestine/Bladder

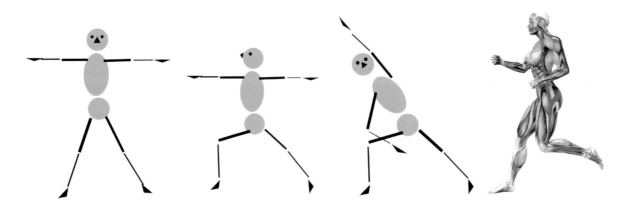

Shao Yang
Triple Warmer/Gall Bladder

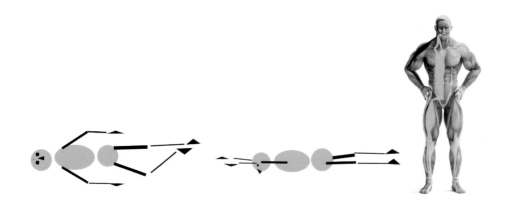

Yang Ming
Large Intestine/Stomach

General Instructions

The Yang *JingJin* run along the back of the body and the outside of the limbs.

Small Intestine/Bladder

Triple Warmer/Gall Bladder

Large Intestine/Stomach

General Instructions:

1. **Start each Yang *JingJin* Stretch from a Neutral Position.**

2. Do Version I of each Yang *JingJin* stretch.

3. Start by holding each stretch to a count of 10. Release.

4. Repeat 3 times.

5. Keep the back and pelvis grounded and anchored.

6. Keep the breath smooth and even. As you exhale, release. As you inhale, open and nourish the fascia and the rest of the body.

7. Gradually increase the repetitions.

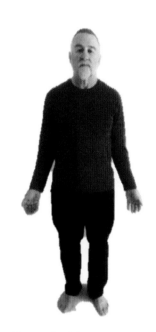

Neutral - Mountain Pose

Version I:

1. Do the stretch sitting in a chair or standing, using the chair for support.

2. If it is difficult to raise the arms or to get up and down from the floor, lie down on an elevated surface, like a bed, sofa, or massage table.

Version II:

• Remove the chair.

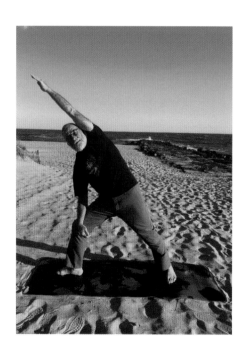

Small Intestine/Bladder – *Tai Yang JingJin*

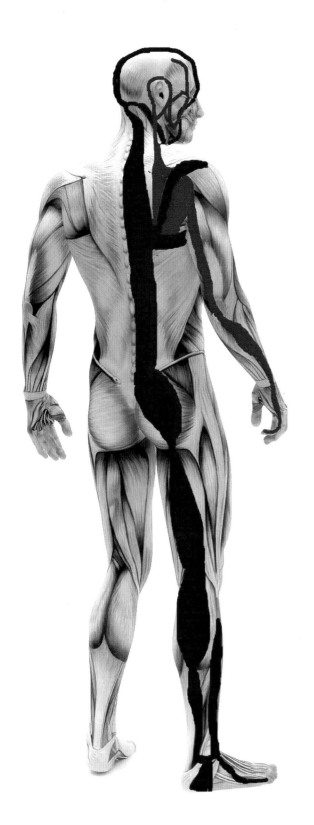

Use this *JingJin* Stretch for:

The immune system, circulation of blood and protective *Qi*. Stiff, strained or twisted muscles, spasms or pain along the *Tai Yang* channels.

Small Intestine: muscles of the little finger, elbow, armpit, arm, back and neck; pain in the elbow, neck, scapula; tinnitus with earache, TMJ syndrome

Bladder: muscles of the little toe and heel, the joints, the spine, armpit or collarbone; inability to raise the arm at the shoulder ("frozen shoulder")

For these Muscles

Little finger and wrist: abductor & extensor digiti minimi, extensor carpi ulnaris

Arm, Shoulder & Neck: anconeus, triceps, teres minor, infraspinatus, rhomboids, serratus posterior superior, splenius cervices & capitis, levator scapulae, sternocleidomastoid, scalenes

Face & Head: orbicularis oculi, occipitalis, frontalis, semispinalis capitis

Legs: hamstrings, gastrocnemius

Back: erector spinae, intrinsic muscles of the spine (rotatores, multifidus, semispinalis), latissimus dorsi, quadratus lumborum, posterior intercostals

Tai Yang JingJin Stretch

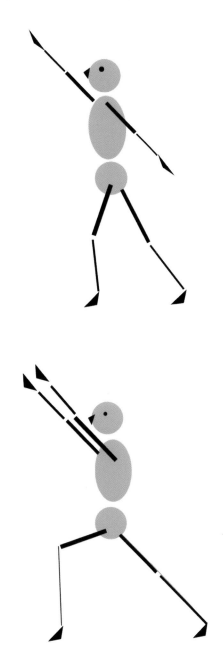

Warrior I

Virabhadrasana

Virabhadra = Warrior, Asana = Pose

(veer-ah-bah-DRAHS-anna)

Tai Yang JingJin Stretch
Version I

1. The instructions will be for the *left* side of your body. You will repeat on the *right*. Place a chair at the end of the short side of your yoga mat. Stand in Mountain Pose (neutral) facing the chair.

2. **Before you begin moving, *imagine* the feeling of a string of fascia running along the meridian, connecting your *left* little finger and *left* little toe.** Imagine stretching the string by pulling the ends away from each other. Maintain this awareness throughout the stretch.

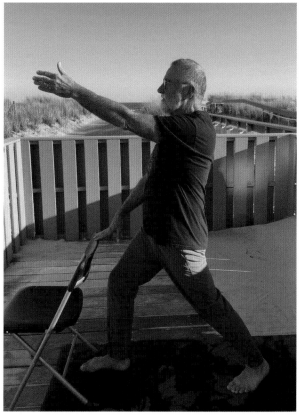

3. Stabilize yourself with your *right* hand on the back of the chair and take one step back with the *left* foot. Adjust your back foot for stability at a distance that is comfortable for you. Square your hips, with your feet parallel as though on a railroad track.

4. Bend your right knee over your ankle, right shin perpendicular to the floor. Detect a lengthening in your back *left* leg all the way to your *left* toe.

5. Raise your *left* arm approximately 45 degrees, and extend it until you sense a stretch in the left little finger. Keep your torso, neck and head erect in one long line. Look straight ahead, create space in the back of your neck and notice a gentle stretch. Soften your gaze.

6. Bring your awareness to lengthening from *left* little toe up the back of your leg, up your spine to your shoulder blade, the back of your neck and to your left little finger. Play with the connection as you lengthen through the fingers and toes. Hold for a count of 6 (gradually working up to 10) as you deepen your breath. Sense how your abdomen moves as you breathe.

7. Release and return to Mountain Pose (neutral). Lower your gaze and notice the release.

8. Gradually increase the holding time.

9. Repeat steps 1 – 8 on other side by switching *left* and *right* in the instructions.

Version II

- Follow the same sequence without the chair and bring both arms up to 45 degrees, palms facing each other.

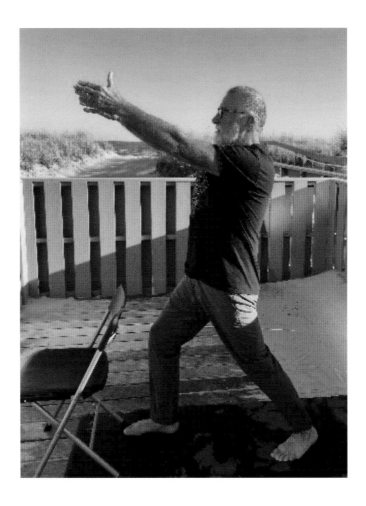

Triple Warmer/Gall Bladder – *Shao Yang JingJin*

Use this *JingJin* Stretch for:

The immune system, circulation of blood and protective *Qi*. Stiff, strained or twisted muscles, spasms or pain along the *Shao Yang* channels, difficulty turning the neck, opening the jaw or raising the arm; improving the circulation of the blood & *Wei Qi*.

Triple Warmer: muscles of the ring finger, elbow, arm, shoulder, neck, jaw and tongue.

Gall Bladder: muscles of the 4th toe, knee (inability to bend or extend), side of the rib cage, breast, clavicle, neck, and those extending from the sacrum upward to below the ribs; muscles of the eyes.

For These Muscles

Head: pterygoids, temporalis, masseter, sternocleidomastoid

Shoulder: supraspinatus, levator scapulae

Hand and Arm: 2-4 interosseous, extensor digitorum

Chest: intercostals

Back & Sides: quadratus lumborum, abdominal obliques, serratus anterior

Leg & Thigh: peroneus (fibularis), iliotibial band, quadratus femoris

Hips: tensor fascia lata, gluteus maximus, minimus, medius, hip rotators (gemellus, obturator, piriformis)

Foot: abductor digiti minimi

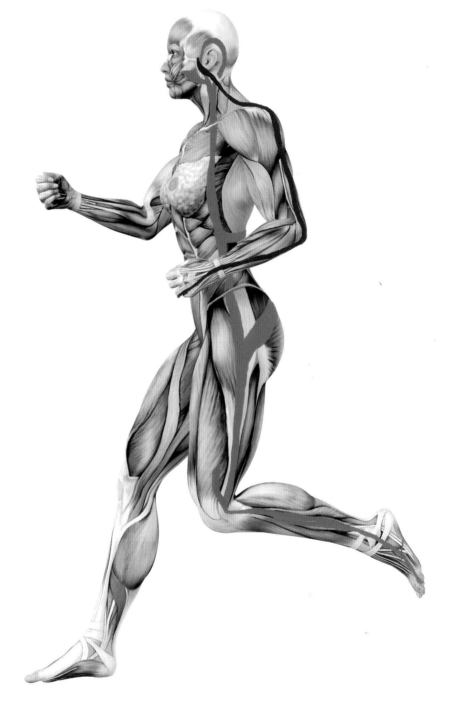

Shao Yang JingJin Stretch

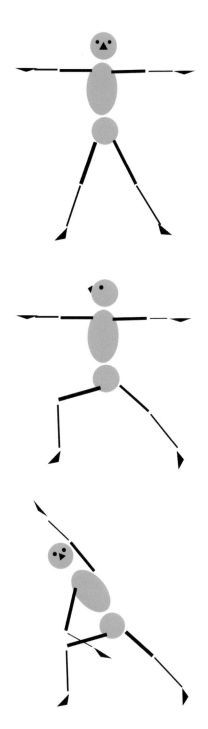

Warrior II/Side Angle

Virabhadrasana II to *Utthita Parsvakonasana*

Virabhadra = Warrior II, *Utthita* = stretched, *parsva* = side, *kona* = angle, *Asana* = Pose

(Veer-ah-bah-DRAHS-anna to oo-TEE-tah parsh-vah-cone-AHS-anna)

Shao Yang JingJin Stretch Version I

1. Instructions are for the *left* side. You will repeat on the *right*. Place a chair on your *right*. Stand in Mountain Pose (neutral) on the mat with your *right* side next to the chair, facing the long side of the mat. **Before you begin moving, *imagine* the feeling of a string of fascia running along the meridian, connecting your *left* ring (4th) finger and 4th *left* toe.** Imagine stretching the string by pulling the ends away from each other. Maintain this awareness throughout the stretch.

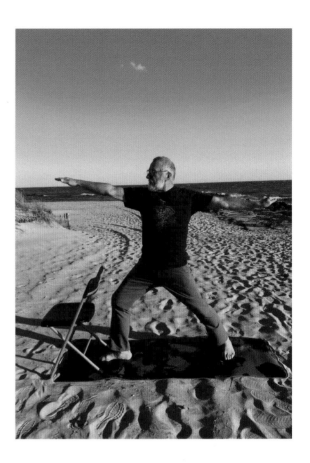

2. Spread your feet a little wider than hip width apart. Square up your hips and then turn the *right* foot (next to the chair) so that the toes are facing it and turn the *left* foot slightly toward the same direction. As you do the stretch find the distance between your feet that is comfortable for you.

3. Extend your arms out to the sides, palms down, parallel to the floor. Reach fingertip to fingertip, ring finger of one hand to ring finger of other hand, engaging the back of the wrist, the elbow, the shoulder and the side of the neck.

4. Release arms to the side. Bend the *right* knee. Keep your knee over your ankle to support joint over joint. The shin is perpendicular to the floor.

5. Keep your hips facing the long edge of the mat, keep your torso, neck and head in a straight line as you lean to the *right*. Lengthen through your *left* ribcage and waist as you lower your *right* hand to rest on the chair for support. Soften your shoulders.

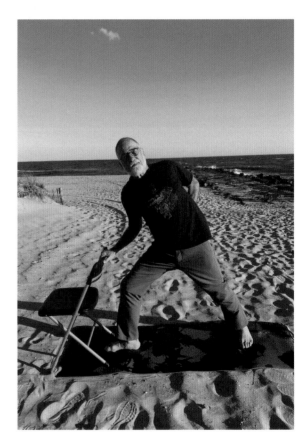

6. Bring your *left* arm to your *left* hip or behind your back if that's comfortable. Feel the stretch on the *left* side of your body through your torso, under your armpit and the side of your neck. Keeping

your neck long, lengthen through the crown of your head. Let your gaze drop to the floor if you have discomfort. Sense the connection between ring finger and 4th toe.

7. Then, as far as is comfortable, lift the *left arm* towards the ceiling with a soft elbow, then gradually form a straight line with your *left leg* as you sense the stretch between *left* ring finger and *left* 4th toe.

8. Start by holding for a count of 6 (increasing to 10) as you deepen your breath in your abdomen. Sense how your abdomen moves as you breathe. Soften the stretch. Release and return to Mountain Pose (neutral). Lower your gaze and notice the release.

9. Repeat steps 1-6 on other side by switching *left* and *right* in the instructions.

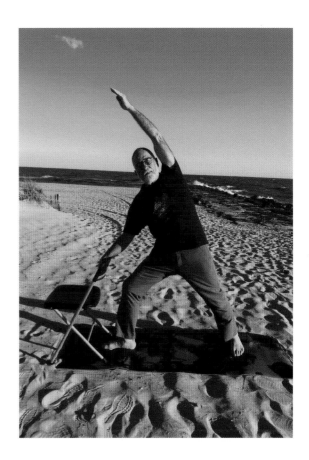

Version II

- Do steps 1 through 9 as in Version I. Release the chair, resting the *right forearm* on your thigh. Then raise your *left arm* up, to reach alongside your ear, forming a straight line with your *left leg*. Repeat, *right*.

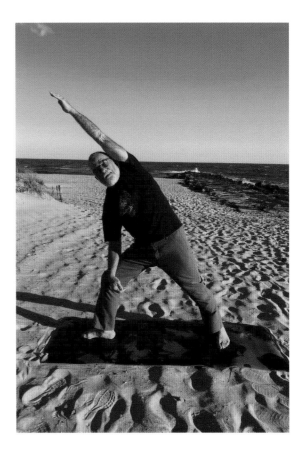

Large Intestine/Stomach – *Yang Ming JingJin*

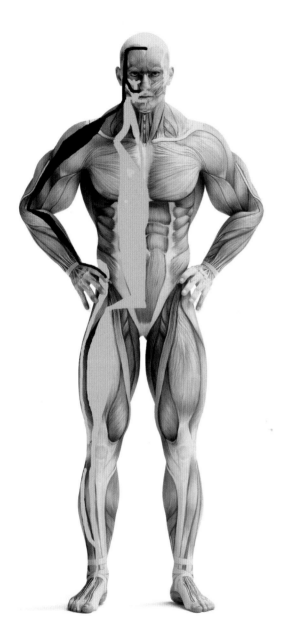

Use this *JingJin* Stretch for:

The immune system: circulation of blood and protective Qi. Stiff, strained or twisted muscles, spasms and pain along the *Yang Ming* channels.

Large Intestine: muscles of the index finger, inability to raise the arm at the shoulder (abduction), pain in the fingers, inability to rotate the neck from side to side.

Stomach: muscles of the middle toe and foot; lateral foot drop; hernia; abdominal muscles, muscles of the neck and cheek, jaw; stretches the deep hip flexors of the pelvis, as well as the front of the thighs; important for proper alignment of the pelvis.

For These Muscles

Neck, Jaw & Face: all hyoids, digastric, mentalis, depressor labii inferior, orbicularis oris, buccinator, risorius, zygomaticus major & minor, levator labii superioris, levator anguli oris, orbicularis oculi

Hand & Arm: extensor pollicis longus & brevis, abductor pollicis longus, extensor carpi radialis, brachioradialis

Shoulder & Neck: deltoid, trapezius, platysma, scalenes

Abdomen: rectus abdominus, external & internal obliques, transversus abdominus

Foot, Leg & Thigh: interosseous, extensor digitorum, tibialis anterior, extensor hallucis, quadriceps, sartorius

Yang Ming JingJin Stretch

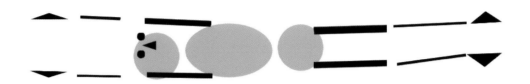

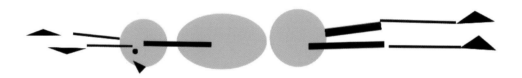

Locust Pose

Salabhasana

Salabha = Locust, *Asana* = Pose

(Sha-la-bhA-sa-na)

Yang Ming JingJin Stretch
Version I

1. Lie on your back on the floor or bed, arrange support under your head and knees if necessary. Begin in neutral with your arms by your sides, legs hip width apart and toes pointing toward the ceiling. **Before you begin moving, *imagine the feeling of a string of fascia running along the meridian, connecting your index finger and 2nd toe** *on the same side*.** Imagine stretching the string by pulling the ends away from each other. Maintain this awareness throughout the stretch.

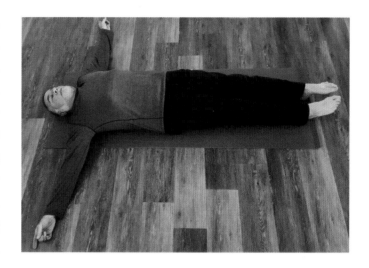

2. *Point your index fingers* as you make a *gentle fist*. Extend your arms out perpendicular to your body to form a T, palms up.

3. While continuing to lengthen through your *index fingers*, point your toes towards the floor.

4. Play with the connection, as you lengthen through the fingers and toes. Hold for a count of 6 (increasing gradually to 10) as you deepen your breath in your abdomen. Sense how your abdomen moves as you breathe. Soften the stretch.

5. Release to neutral. Bring your arms in and hug your knees to your chest. Close your eyes and notice the release. Gradually increase the time.

Version II

- Do steps one through 3 as in Version I. Bring the arms overhead as far as is comfortable, palms up, knuckles facing each other and toes pointed. Extend the stretch.

- Continue with steps 4 and 5.

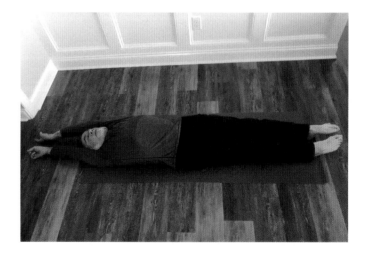

Version III

1. Begin by turning over and lying flat on your abdomen. As you take a breath, feel your legs extended behind you, hip width apart. Place your forehead on the mat, neck long and arms stretched overhead. Slightly rotate the palms towards the outside, index finger extended. Imagine the string connecting the **index finger and 2nd toe**.

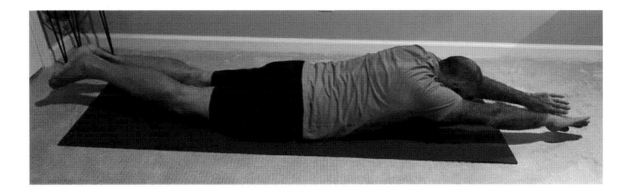

2. Inhale into the abdomen. Engage your abdominal muscles as you lift the arms, head, chest and legs off the floor, lengthening through the arms and legs. Allow your arms and legs to float gently up and down with the breath.

   TIP: the key is length, not lift.

3. Press back into the child pose and rest.

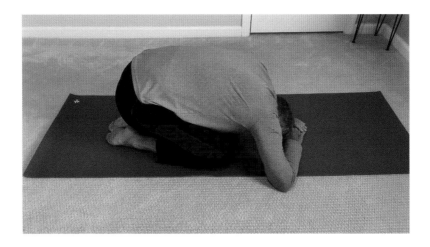

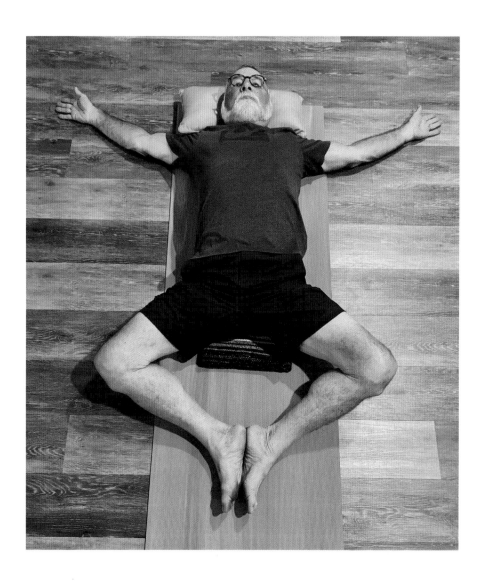

Chapter Six:
Yin *JingJin* Stretches

As You Begin:

Remember, the goal is awareness of your body.

Be patient with yourself and stay in the present moment.

Begin with **Version I** of the stretch.

Go slow, breathe, take it easy.

Remember the balance of Yin and Yang:

Start at 75% of what you think you can do. Look for your edge and stay just on the comfortable side of it, where you feel that satisfying stretch without excessive discomfort or pain. Let your body tell you when it's ready to extend the stretch.

Breathing: Before starting the stretch, exhale to empty. During the stretch, *inhale* **as you lengthen,** *exhale* **as you release** and open the fascia.

The *release* is the important part.

Golden Rule:
Less Is More!

THE YIN *JINGJIN* RUN ALONG THE FRONT OF THE BODY AND THE INSIDES OF THE LIMBS.

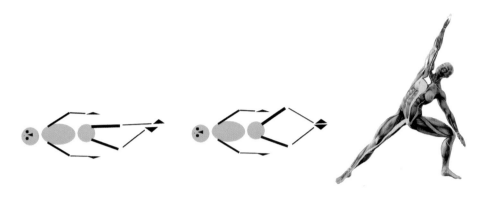

Lung/Spleen

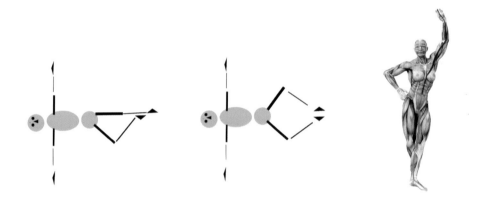

Jue Yin
Pericardium/Liver

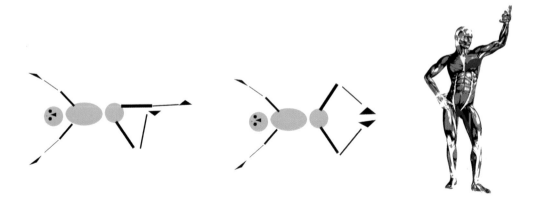

Shao Yin
Heart/Kidney

Yin *JingJin* Stretches

Yin *JingJin* run along the front of the body and the insides of the limbs.
Lung/Spleen
Heart/Kidney
Pericardium/Liver

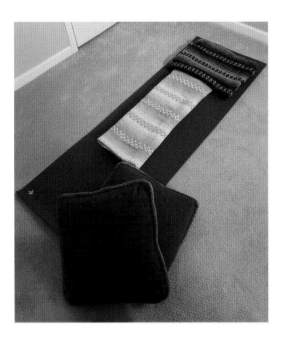

Props

Blankets for under the spine to open the torso.
Pillows and/or blocks under the knees for support.

General Instructions

1. **Start each Yin *JingJin* Stretch in Neutral Position.**

2. Use added pillows and blankets as needed.

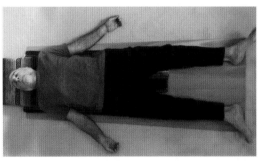

3. Start by holding each stretch for five minutes.

4. Keep the back and pelvis grounded and anchored.

5. Keep the breath smooth and even. As you exhale, release. As you inhale, open and nourish the fascia and the rest of the body.

6. Gradually extend your stay anywhere from five to ten minutes.

Version I

1. Lie down on an elevated surface, like a bed, sofa, or massage table with a yoga mat under your feet.

2. If it is difficult to lie down, do the stretch sitting in a chair

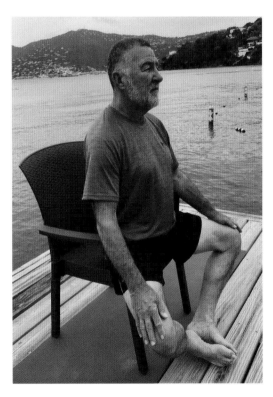

Lung/Spleen – *Tai Yin JingJin*

Use this *JingJin* Stretch for:

The immune system: circulation of blood and protective Qi. Stiff, strained or twisted muscles, spasms and pain along the course of the *Tai Yin* channels

Lung: muscles of the thumb, anterior arm; muscle spasms over the ribs

Spleen: muscles of the big toe, inner anklebone, inside of the knee, thigh adductors, groin, upper abdominals, mid-thoracic intercostals, genitalia

For These Muscles

Fingers, Hand & Arm: abductor, flexor, opponens, adductor pollicis muscles, biceps, brachialis, anterior deltoid, coracobrachialis

Chest: pectoralis major & minor, upper diaphragm

Abdomen: iliopsoas, lower diaphragm

Foot, Leg & Thigh: abductor hallucis, tibialis posterior, adductors of the thigh

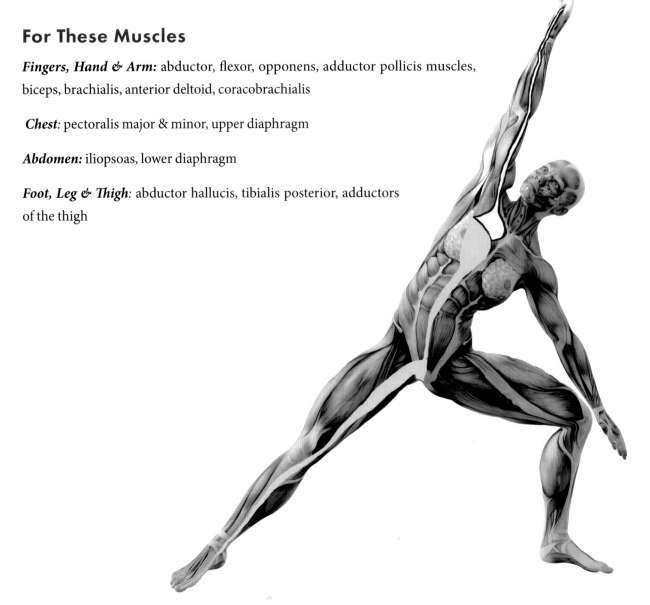

Tai Yin JingJin Stretch

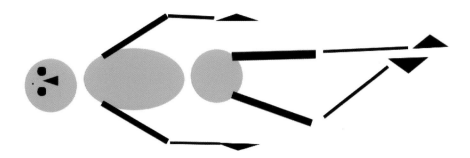

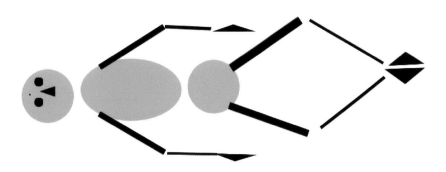

Reclining Bound Angle I

Supta Baddha Konasana

Supta = lying down supine, *Baddha* = bound, *Kona* = angle, *asana* = pose

(*Soup-tah BAH-dah-cone-NAHS-anna*)

Tai Yin JingJin Stretch
Version I

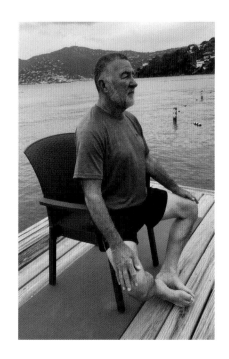

1. Sitting in a sturdy chair, bring the soles of your feet together, and allow the knees to relax and open as far as is comfortable. **Before you begin moving, *imagine* the feeling of a string of fascia running along the meridian, connecting your *thumbs and inside of your big toes* (medial) on the same side.** Imagine the feeling of stretching the string by pulling the ends away from each other. Maintain this awareness throughout the stretch.

2. Bring your hands out to the side, extend the thumbs with the palms facing forward.

Version II

1. Sitting on a mat on the floor (or bed), arrange a blanket under your torso from head to tailbone to open the chest, and a pillow next to each knee. Lower onto your back with a thin pillow or blanket roll under your head and neck for support. **Before you begin moving, imagine the feeling of a string connecting your *thumbs and the inside of your big toes* on the same side.** Imagine the feeling of stretching the string by pulling the ends away from each other. Maintain this awareness throughout the stretch.

2. Keeping both shoulders on the floor and using the props for your knees, bend the right knee and bring the sole of the foot to the *opposite (left) ankle*.

    Then bring the *opposite (left) heel up to meet the right*, flexing the ankles and reaching through the *big toes*. Adjust the pillows under the knees for comfort. Less is more.

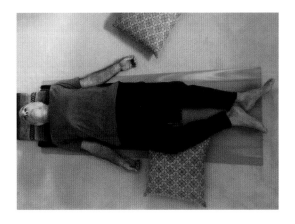 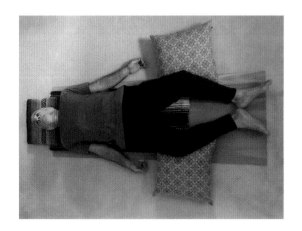

3. Resting your hands on your torso or the top of your thighs, imagine the feeling of your knees floating up toward the ceiling and continue settling deep into your pelvis. As your pelvis releases toward the floor, so will your knees. Feel the spine lengthening and the chest opening. Bring awareness up the body on **both sides** at the same time, starting from the *big toes* through the inside of the knees, inner thighs, pelvis, moving out toward the sides of the ribcage, then out the inside of the arms to the *thumbs*.

4. Release the arms to lie alongside the body. Then extend your thumbs with palm side up, feeling the stretch from the inside of the *big toes* through the front of shoulder through the inside of the arm to the *thumbs on the same side*. Soften into the position for one minute, as you hold the stretch. Deepen your breath in your abdomen, sense how your abdomen moves as you breathe. Gradually extend your stay anywhere from five to ten minutes.

5. Bring your knees up to your chest, then roll over onto one side and rest. Notice the release before coming into a sitting position.

Version III

- Do Version II, then slowly remove the supports from under your knees.

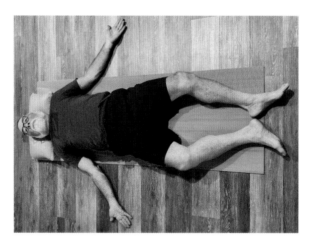

Note: The natural tendency is to push the knees toward the floor to increase the stretch of the inner thighs and groin. But, especially if the groin is tight, pushing the knees down will have just the **opposite** *of the intended effect. The groin will harden, as will the belly and lower back of the inner thighs and groin.*

Pericardium/Liver – *Jue Yin JingJin*

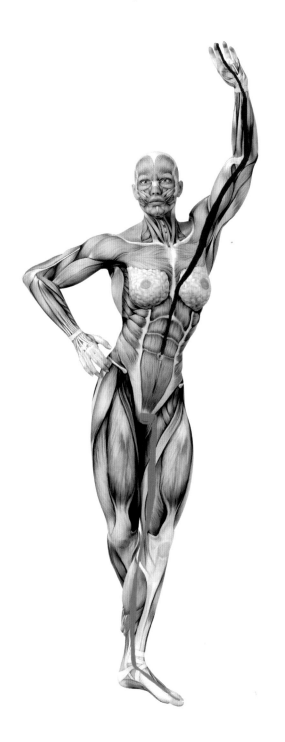

Use this *JingJin* Stretch for:

The immune system: circulation of blood and protective Qi. Stiff, strained or twisted muscles, spasm and pain along the course of the *Jue Yin* channels

Pericardium: muscles of the middle finger, palm, inside of the arm, chest

Liver: muscles of the big toe, inside ankle, medial knee, medial thigh, the genitals

For These Muscles

Hand & Arm: palmar interosseous, lumbricales, pronator quadratus, pronator teres, flexor carpi radialis, palmaris longus, flexor digitorum, superficialis & profundus, brachialis

Shoulder: lattisimus dorsi, teres major, subscapularis, serratus anterior

Chest: intercostals, diaphragm

Foot, Leg & Thigh: flexor & adductor hallucis, extensor digitorum longus, adductor brevis

Jue Yin JingJin Stretch

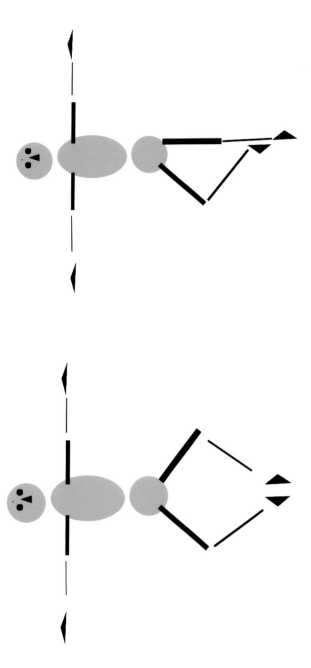

Reclining Bound Angle II

Supta Baddha Konasana

Supta = lying down supine, Baddha = bound, Kona = angle, *asana* = pose

(*Soup-tah BAH-dah-cone-NAHS-anna*)

Jue Yin JingJin Stretch
Version I

1. Sitting in a sturdy chair, bring the soles of your feet together, and allow the knees to relax and open as far as is comfortable for you. **Before you begin moving,** *imagine* **the feeling of a string of fascia running along the meridian, connecting your** *middle fingers* **and** *outside (lateral side) of your big toes*. Imagine the feeling of stretching the string by pulling the ends away from each other. Maintain this awareness throughout the stretch.

2. Bring your hands out to the side at shoulder level (or as far up as you can), extend the middle finger with the palms facing forward.

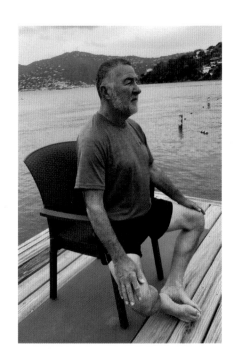

Version II

1. Sitting on a mat on the floor (or bed), arrange a blanket under your torso from head to tailbone to open the chest, and a pillow next to each knee. Lower onto your back with a thin pillow or blanket roll under your head and neck for support. **Before you begin moving, imagine the feeling of a string connecting your** *middle fingers* **and the** *outside of your big toes on the same side*. *Imagine* the feeling of stretching the string by pulling the ends away from each other. Maintain this awareness throughout the stretch.

2. Keeping both shoulders on the floor and using the props for your knees, bend the *left knee* and bring the sole of that *foot* to the *opposite (right) calf.*

   Then bring the *opposite (right) heel up to meet the first*, flexing the ankle and reaching through the *outside of your big toes.* Adjust the pillows under the knees for comfort. Less is more.

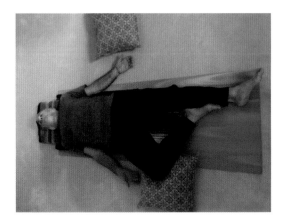 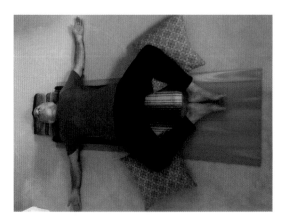

3.   Resting your hands on your torso or the top of your thighs, imagine the feeling of your knees floating up toward the ceiling and continue settling deep into your pelvis. As your pelvis releases toward the floor, so will your knees. Feel the spine lengthening and the chest opening. Release the arms and extend them to a T, palms up, as far as is comfortable for you. Bring awareness up the body on **both sides** at the same time, starting from the outside of the *big toes through the* inside of the knees, inner thighs, pelvis, front of the torso to the bottom of the rib cage, up the chest and out the inside of the arms to the *middle fingers*. Soften into the position for one minute as you hold the stretch. Deepen your breath in your abdomen, sense how your abdomen moves as you breathe. Gradually extend your stay anywhere from 5 to 10 minutes.

4.   Bring your knees to your chest, then roll over onto one side and rest. Notice the release before coming into a sitting position.

Version III

- Do the steps in Version III, slowly removing the supports under the knees.

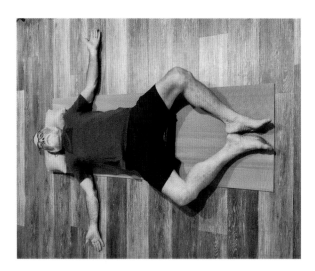

Note: The natural tendency in this stretch is to push the knees toward the floor to increase the stretch of the inner thighs and pelvis. But especially if the pelvis is tight, pushing the knees down will have just the ***opposite*** *of the intended effect. The pelvic muscles will harden, as will the belly and lower back.*

Heart/Kidney –*Shao Yin JingJin*

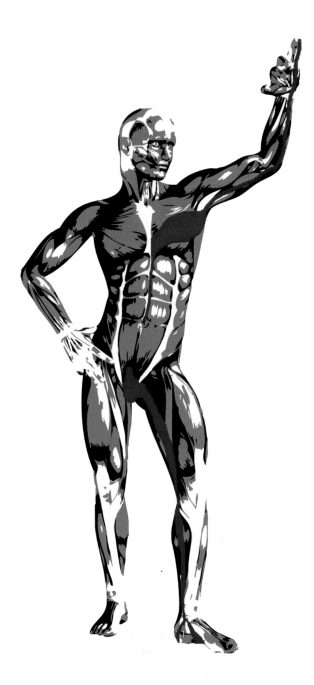

Use this *JingJin* Stretch for:

Support for the immune system: circulation of blood and protective Qi. Stiff, strained or twisted muscles, spasms or pain along the *Shao Yin* channels

Heart: muscles of the little finger, speech difficulties, feeling of fullness in the chest, internal cramping sensation (like object stuck in chest)

Kidney: muscles of the bottom of the foot, pain in the groin (especially shooting down the thigh toward the inside ankle bone), difficulty extending or flexing the neck and/or back; low back pain; the knee, inner thigh and groin

For These Muscles

Hand, Forearm & Arm: opponens & flexor digiti minimi, flexors of the arm, biceps

Chest: pectoralis major (lower fibers)

Pelvis: levator ani, coccyx

Spine: intrinsic rotators (rotatores, multifidus)

Foot, Leg & Thigh: plantar interosseous, lumbricales, flexor digitorum longus & brevis, adductor magnus, gracilis

Shao Yin JingJin Stretch

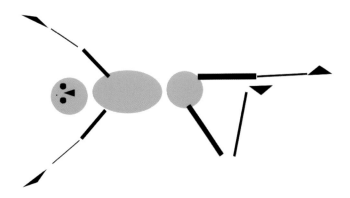

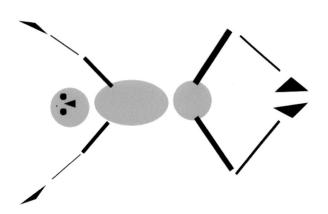

Reclining Bound Angle III

Supta Baddha Konasana

Supta = lying down supine, *Baddha* = bound, *Kona* = angle, *asana* = pose

(*Soup-tah BAH-dah-cone-NAHS-anna*)

Shao Yin JingJin Stretch
Version I

1. Sitting in a sturdy chair, bring the soles of your feet together, and allow the knees to relax and open as far as is comfortable for you. **Before you begin moving,** *imagine* **the feeling** of **a string of fascia running along the meridian, connecting your *(little) fingers and (little) toes.*** *Imagine* the feeling of stretching the string by pulling the ends away from each other. Maintain this awareness throughout the stretch.

2. Release your arms to your side, palms up, and move them up beside the body, through a T, toward a Y, until you feel the stretch in the little fingers.

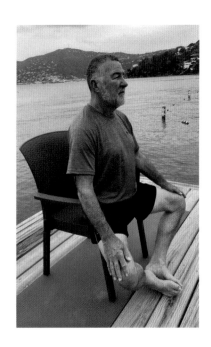

Version II

1. Sitting on a mat on the floor (or bed), arrange a blanket under your torso from head to tailbone to open the chest, and a pillow next to each knee. Lower onto your back with a thin pillow or blanket roll under your head and neck for support. **Before you begin moving,** *imagine* **the feeling of a string connecting your *little fingers and little toes on the same side.*** *Imagine* the feeling of stretching the string by pulling the ends away from each other. Maintain this awareness throughout the stretch.

2. Keeping both shoulders on the floor using the props for your knees, bend *the right knee* and bring the sole of the *foot as close as possible to the opposite (left) knee.*

   Then bring the *opposite (left) heel up to meet the first,* flexing the ankle and reaching through the *little toes.* Adjust the pillows under the knees for support. Less is more.

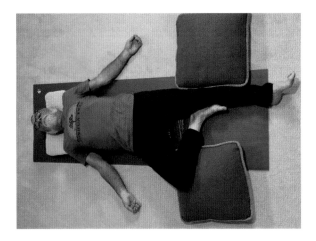
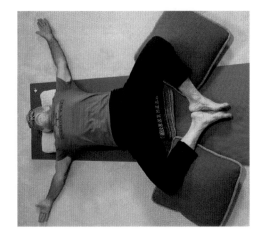

3. Resting your hands on the top of your thighs, imagine the feeling of your knees floating up toward the ceiling and continue settling deep into your pelvis. As your pelvis releases toward the floor, so will your knees. Feel the spine lengthening and the chest opening. Release your arms to your side, palms up and, *keeping them on the floor*, move through a T, toward a Y, until you feel the stretch in the little fingers. Bring awareness up the body on **both sides** at the same time, starting from *little toes* across the soles of the feet to inside the heels, inner knees, thighs, pelvis, diaphragm, up the chest, and out the inside of the arms to the *little fingers*, imagining the string connecting your *little fingers* and *little toes*. Stretch the ends away from each other and at the same time, stretch up the spine from the tailbone to the back of your neck at the base of the skull. Soften into the position for one minute as you hold the stretch. Deepen your breath in your abdomen, sense how your abdomen moves as you breathe. Gradually extend your stay anywhere from five to ten minutes.

4. To come out, bring your knees toward your chest, then roll over onto one side and rest. Notice the release before coming into a sitting position.

Version III

- Do Version II, slowly removing the supports under your knees.

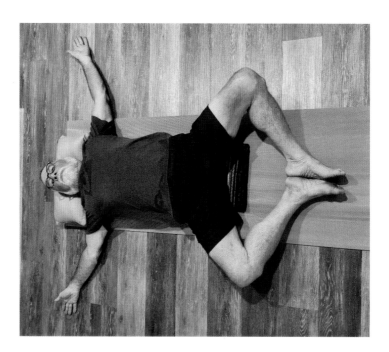

Appendix I:
Sequence Review

Version I and Version II

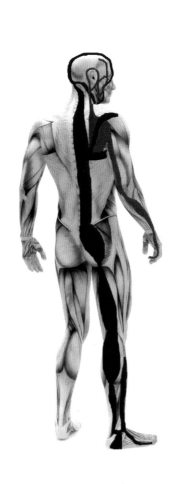
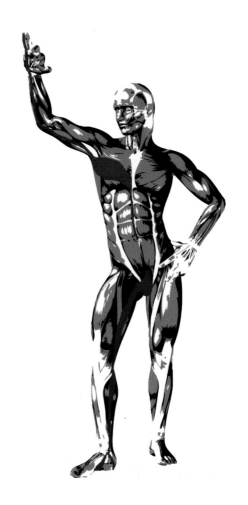

SEQUENCE REVIEW

JingJin Stretches - Version I

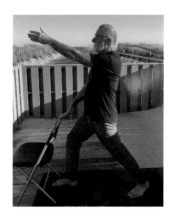

Small Intestine/Bladder
Tai Yang JingJin Stretch
Warrior I

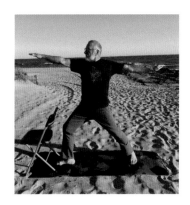 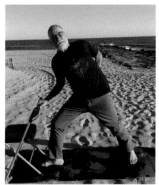 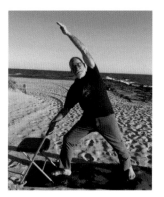

Triple Warmer/Gallbladder
Shao Yang JingJin Stretch
Warrior II to Side Angle

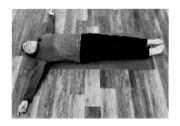 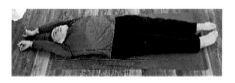

Large Intestine/Stomach
Yang Ming JingJin Stretch
Locust I

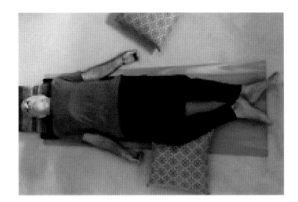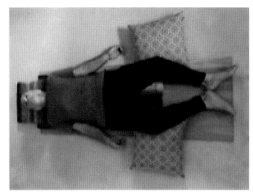

Lung/Spleen
Tai Yin JingJin **Stretch**
Reclining Bound Angle I

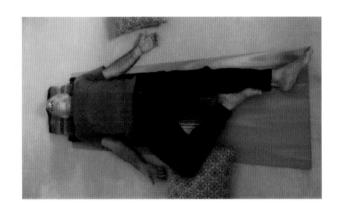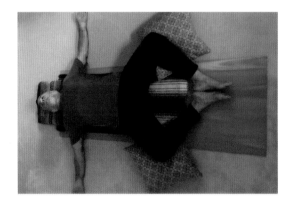

Pericardium/Liver
Jue Yin JingJin **Stretch**
Reclining Bound Angle II

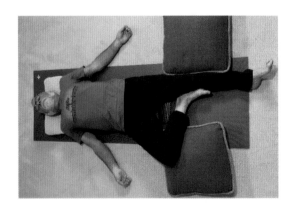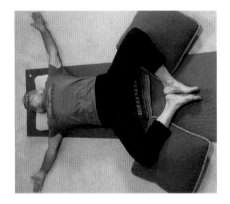

Heart/Kidney
Shao Yin JingJin **Stretch**
Reclining Bound Angle III

SEQUENCE REVIEW
JingJin Stretches - Version II

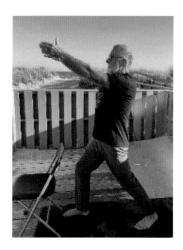

Small Intestine/Bladder
Tai Yang JingJin Stretch
Warrior I

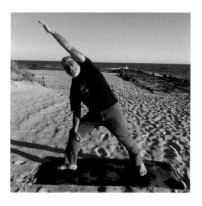

Triple Warmer/Gallbladder
Shao Yang JingJin Stretch
Warrior II to Side Angle

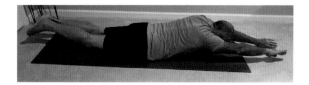

Large Intestine/Stomach
Yang Ming JingJin Stretch
Locust I

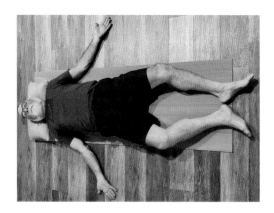

Lung/Spleen
Tai Yin JingJin **Stretch**
Reclining Bound Angle I

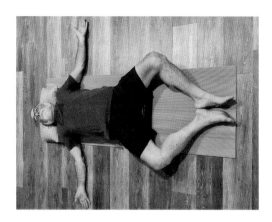

Pericardium/Liver
Jue Yin JingJin **Stretch**
Reclining Bound Angle II

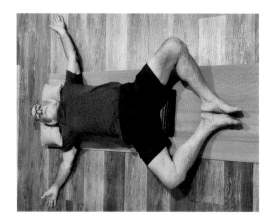

Heart/Kidney
Shao Yin JingJin **Stretch**
Reclining Bound Angle III

Appendix II:
Traditional Chinese Medicine

The Principal Channels

The most commonly used energy pathways for treatment in Chinese Medicine are the principal meridians, which Western translators named after the organs they nourish, e.g. Lung, Stomach, Heart, etc. Their function is much broader than this, however, because, among other things, they each govern aspects of the physiology all the way down to the cell. They are also organized into functional Yin/Yang pairs that have complementary functions and travel through the same area of the body. They are responsible for the major senses, tissues, body fluids, the body's physiological response to climate and the emotions that engage relevant tissues and physiological functions. For instance, the Lung/Large Intestine pair govern elimination, the thumb side of the arm, the skin, mucous, and the emotion of grief. The *JingJin* are branches going to the muscles along the pathways of the principal meridians. As they carry the *Wei Qi* or defensive energy, they form a layer of protective armor that prevents invasion of pathogenic factors.

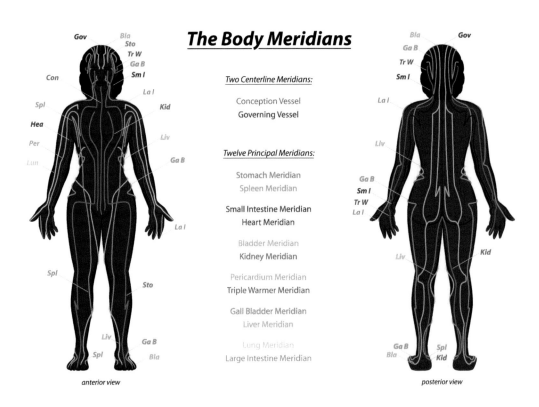

The Body Meridians

Two Centerline Meridians:

Conception Vessel
Governing Vessel

Twelve Principal Meridians:

Stomach Meridian
Spleen Meridian

Small Intestine Meridian
Heart Meridian

Bladder Meridian
Kidney Meridian

Pericardium Meridian
Triple Warmer Meridian

Gall Bladder Meridian
Liver Meridian

Lung Meridian
Large Intestine Meridian

anterior view

posterior view

62

The *JingJin* Channels

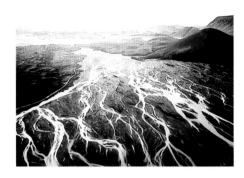

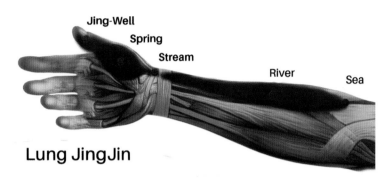

The *JingJin* are related to the principal meridians like deltas are related to rivers. They are more superficial branches that create broad zones in the fascia to nourish muscles, tendons, and ligaments and form a protective layer of *Wei Qi*. Each of these superficial channels comes to the surface from one of the 12 principal meridians at the *Jing-Well* points on the fingers and toes and flows toward the torso. There are five points between the fingertips and elbows and the toes and knees named "Well," "Spring," "Stream," "River" and "Sea" that describe the spreading and building nature of the channels.

Yin and Yang are dynamic, complementary, interdependent opposites. The Chinese characters for Yin and Yang depict the dark side and light side of a mountain that are constantly shifting in the course of a day. At sunrise, the East is light and the West is dark. At sunset, the opposite is true.

So Yin and Yang are relative, not absolute qualities. They exist in relationship to each other and one cannot be perceived without the other. How would we know about light if we've never experienced the dark? The changing recombination and balance between them is what creates the "10,000 things."

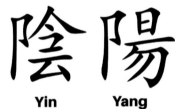

Some of these pairs of complementary opposites are:

YIN	YANG
Dark	Light
Receptive	Active
Structure	Function
Matter	Energy
Negative Pole	Positive Pole
Cool	Warm
Damp	Dry
Anatomy: Front of Torso and Inside of Limbs	Anatomy: The Head, Back of Torso and Outside of Limbs

Appendix III:
Link to *JingJin* Yoga Videos

Links to videos of the six *JingJin* stretches:

Jue Yin JingJin Yoga Stretch
https://youtu.be/xOexILH6NsQ

Shao Yin JingJin Yoga Stretch
https://youtu.be/aJfKe3MqQ8s

Tai Yin JingJin Yoga Stretch
https://youtu.be/6JZsvttGzm0

Yang Ming JingJin Yoga Stretch
https://youtu.be/5uQ3B7Xc0U4

Tai Yang JingJin Yoga Stretch
https://youtu.be/9t0esV84Pqw

Shao Yang JingJin Yoga Stretch
https://youtu.be/nCc6EPYjVtI

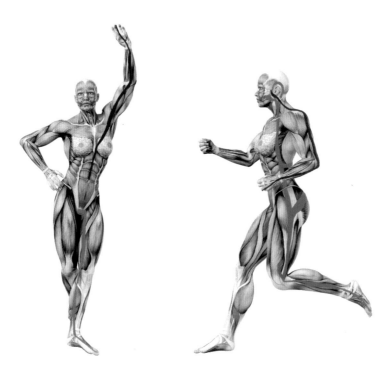

Bibliography

Anderson, Sandra, and Rolf Sovik, *Yoga, Mastering the Basics*. Honesdale, PA, Himalayan Institute Press, 2000.

Coulter, H. David, *Anatomy of Hatha Yoga*, Honesdale, PA, Body and Breath, 2001.

Ellis, Andrew, Wiseman, Nigel, and Boss, Ken. *Fundamentals of Chinese Acupuncture*, Brookline, MA, Paradigm Publications, 1991.

Legge, David, *Jing Jin: Acupuncture treatment of the muscular system using the meridian sinews*, Journal of Chinese Medicine, Publishers, 1/1/10.

Maciocia, Giovanni, *The Foundations of Chinese Medicine,* Churchill Livingston, 1996.

Shanghai College of Traditional Medicine, *Acupuncture, A Comprehensive Text*, 1981, Eastland Press, Seattle.

Smith, Deborah Valentine; *North American Journal of Oriental Medicine,* "Tendinomuscular Meridians," 2010.

Solinas, Henri; Auteroche, Bernard and Mainville, Lucie, *Atlas D'Acupuncture Chinoise, 1. Topographie des meridiens,"* Editions Maloine, Paris, 1990.

The Journal of Chinese Medicine, The Five Shu Points, No. 42 May 1993. https://www.journalofchinesemedicine.com/the-five-shupoints.html

Tseng et.al, *International Journal of Nursing and Clinical Practice,* 2015, 2:12. http://dx.doi.org/10.15344/2394-4978/2015/121

Related Internet Links

For videos of all six *JingJin* Stretches, subscribe to *JingJin Yoga* at
https://www.youtube.com/@jingjinyoga

Hedley, Gil, Fascia and Stretching: "The Fuzz Speech"
https://www.youtube.com/watch?v=_FtSP-tkSug

Clarey, Christopher; Olympians Use Imagery as Mental Training.
https://www.nytimes.com/2014/02/23/sports/olympics/olympians-use-imagery-as-mental-training.html

Falkenberg, R.I., Eising, C., and Peters, M.L.; Yoga and Immune System Functioning
https://link.springer.com/article/10.1007/s10865-018-9914-y

Newport Academy, "Understanding the Mind-Body Connection."
https://www.newportacademy.com/resources/mental-health/understanding-the-mind-body-connection/

Qigong for the Tendinomuscular Meridians:
http://www.yoga-taichi91.fr/en_qigong_yi_jing_jin.html

Two-part Article on the *JingJin* by Marty Eisen
http://yang-sheng.com/?p=11087
http://yang-sheng.com/?p=11218

Acknowledgements

WE ARE BLESSED TO HAVE HAD THE HELP OF STUDENTS, COLLEAGUES AND family while we prepared this book and we offer our most heartfelt thanks to each of them. We are especially grateful to John R. Piotrowski who modeled the stretches and endlessly reviewed the text. Caroline Foote's expertise in promotion and editing was invaluable. Thanks also to John S. Piotrowski, Jean Jewell, Pat Beaupre Becker and Donna Huse for pivotal feedback on format and content. Thanks also to Nema Nyar from the Himalayan Institute for review of the manuscript.

We also want to honor the long lineages of teachers who came before us and preserved and passed on these beautiful healing arts for self-discovery, self-healing and self-transformation. In particular our Asian bodywork mentors, Iona Marsaa Teeguarden, M.A., L.M.F.T, AOBTA® Certified Instructor; Sensei Wataru Ohashi, Ruth Dalphin, M.M., L.Ac., and our Yoga mentors, Sandra Anderson, Rolf Sovik, Psy.D., and Shari Friedrichsen.

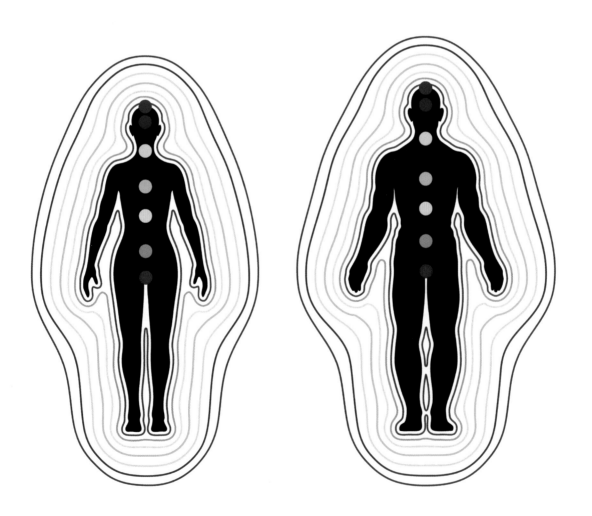

66

Graphics/Photo Credits

Anatomical Diagrams edited by Deborah Valentine Smith:
Tai Yang: Shutterstock 118596400; *Shao Yang*: Shutterstock 11422354086; *Yang Ming*: Shutterstock 247631068;
Tai Yin: Shutterstock 778484293; *Shao Yin*: Shutterstock 115051813; *Jue Yin*: Shutterstock 1197041665

Stick Figures: Deborah Valentine Smith

Asana Photos: Barbara "Teddy" Piotrowski

Yin/Yang Lotus Copyright: www.123rf.com/profile_wasiliymay ID 58795090

Lotus Bud: Photo: Jeshu John

Delta: Photo: pexels.com

Muscle Structure: Copyright: www.123rf.com/profile_tigatelu

Candy: Candy, Garsaya/123RF.com ID 64638082

Muscle Fiber: Design 36/Shutterstock.com ID: 124585756

Sponges: niceregionpics/123RF.com ID 17725880

Boy in Blanket: www.123rf.com/profile_tomsickova ID 137430945

Yoga in the Snow: *New York Times*

Two Heads: Benjavisa Ruangvaree Art/Shutterstock.com ID: 1206995659

Sunrise: Pexels at pixabay/268134

Contentment Diagram: Barbara "Teddy" Piotrowski

Principal Meridians www.123rf.com/profile_peterhermesfurian ID149677380

Lung *JingJin*: Deborah Valentine Smith

Auras: Copyright: www.123rf.com/profile_deosum ID 61444037

Photo of Deborah Valentine Smith by Gerald Sampson

Photo of Teddy Piotrowski by J.C. Penny

About the Authors

Deborah Valentine Smith

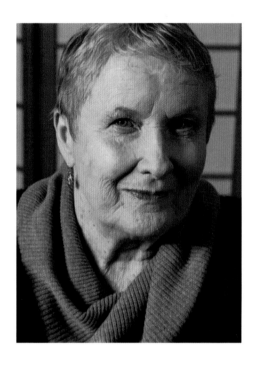

Deborah Valentine Smith, B.A., Dipl. ABT (NCCAOM®), is a Registered Jin Shin Do® Bodymind Acupressure® practitioner (since 1979) and a senior Authorized JSD Teacher (since 1983). She is a licensed massage therapist in New York, board certified and an approved provider with the National Certification Board for Therapeutic Massage and Bodywork (NCBTMB), and a Certified Instructor with the American Organization for Bodywork Therapies of Asia (AOBTA®). She has taught worldwide in massage and bodywork schools, learning centers, and formal training programs.

Deborah is especially interested in teaching self-care techniques to the public and teaches privately wherever people want to learn. She is currently enjoying the evolution of her online course: "Western Body, Eastern Mind: Integrated Anatomy and Physiology," which is accepted as the A&P requirement for Certified AOBTA® Practitioners. She contributed 3 chapters to *A Complete Guide to Acupressure* by Iona Marsaa Teeguarden, M.A., L.M.F.T, served as the Editor-in-Chief of *Pulse*, the newsletter of the AOBTA®, for 16 years, and has published articles on Asian Bodywork Therapies in numerous publications including *Massage Magazine, Acupuncture Today, Massage Today, The North American Journal of Chinese Medicine and* the AOBTA®'s *Pulse*. She has served as president and in many other capacities on the AOBTA® board of directors since its inception in 1989. Deborah sees clients virtually and in New Paltz, New York.

Barbara "Teddy" Piotrowski

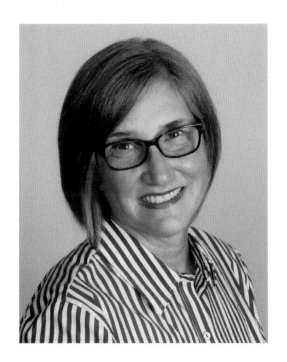

Barbara "Teddy" Piotrowski, RN, HNB-BC, BA, Dipl. ABT (NCCAOM®), C-IAYT is a Board-Certified Holistic Nurse with more than 40 years of medical experience. She is a Certified Yoga Therapist, a Diplomate of Asian Bodywork Therapy, with an expertise in Shiatsu and Acupressure, and has been a Reiki Master, for over 20 years. As a Registered Nurse, Teddy saw the benefits of Eastern healing arts and believed it to be crucial to integrate them into everyday living. The self-care they provide is a piece that was missing in her Western based medical training.

Through the years Teddy has assisted individuals in all stages of life; from children and teens, couples working through fertility concerns, to older adults. Along with her own growth and acceptance of Eastern therapeutic ideals, she nourished the growth of her company, Greater Harmony, a business totally dedicated to promoting the benefits of a healthier and a more energetic way of life.

Working to champion yoga and meditation as healing arts and sciences, Teddy's focus led her to working with the senior population. She empowers individuals to progress toward improved health and well-being through the application of the teachings and practices of yoga. The yoga tradition views each human being as a multidimensional system that encompasses numerous aspects including: body, breath, and mind (intellect and emotions) and their interaction. In 2005, she began working in a Continuing Care Retirement Community, developing a program with the medical director and other health care professionals that provided a safe and effective program for the residents. By understanding the various health problems that older students face, she was able to adapt the postures and movements that are essential to making the practice both safe and effective. Teddy is currently teaching classes privately and for the local county senior health departments.